When Annie Came to Visit

AF697454

When Annie Came to Visit

A Brain Aneurysm Survivor's Journey

KELLI SCHOEN

TATE PUBLISHING
AND ENTERPRISES, LLC

When Annie Came to Visit
Copyright © 2013 by Kelli Schoen. All rights reserved.

No part of this publication may be reproduced, stored in a retrieval system or transmitted in any way by any means, electronic, mechanical, photocopy, recording or otherwise without the prior permission of the author except as provided by USA copyright law.

This book is designed to provide accurate and authoritative information with regard to the subject matter covered. This information is given with the understanding that neither the author nor Tate Publishing, LLC is engaged in rendering legal, professional advice. Since the details of your situation are fact dependent, you should additionally seek the services of a competent professional.

The opinions expressed by the author are not necessarily those of Tate Publishing, LLC.

Published by Tate Publishing & Enterprises, LLC
127 E. Trade Center Terrace | Mustang, Oklahoma 73064 USA
1.888.361.9473 | www.tatepublishing.com

Tate Publishing is committed to excellence in the publishing industry. The company reflects the philosophy established by the founders, based on Psalm 68:11,
"The Lord gave the word and great was the company of those who published it."

Book design copyright © 2013 by Tate Publishing, LLC. All rights reserved.
Cover design by Rtor Maghuyop
Interior design by Deborah Toling
Author photo by Kelsey Thompson Photography

Published in the United States of America

ISBN: 978-1-62854-329-2
1. Biography & Autobiography / Personal Memoirs
2. Biography & Autobiography / General
13.08.05

Contents

Introduction

I decided to write this book when I was told I could not work. This happened after Annie came to visit me. That was when I realized Annie took something major from me. My job was my life. It was, I guess, my purpose in life. I had to come up with a new purpose in my life. Sitting around doing nothing just wasn't cutting it! My new purpose, I decided, was to share my story in hopes that it will help someone else. My story is not special. There are many of us who have been visited by Annie and had our lives turned upside down. I just don't think there is much awareness about Annie. So, I figured by sharing my story I will help spread awareness of Annie. If it helps people in other ways, that's great also. I'm writing as if I'm talking to someone who has been affected by a major health event and had to then take the recovery journey. I am hoping that by sharing my visit from Annie and my recovery journey, I may help you in some way. It is not easy to come back from a major medical event but it can happen. Read my story and see how I have been coming back one step at a time since Annie came to visit me.

Okay. I'll tell you the truth. Annie is not a person. *Annie* is a nickname for a medical condition called aneurysm. My best laymen's description of an aneurysm is that it is a bulge in a blood vessel. Think of a long, thin balloon. If it gets a kink in it, it can cause a bulge. As more air fills the balloon, the bulge grows bigger and bigger until it explodes—that is, unless you see the kink in time and fix it so that all the air can go into the balloon. I went on the Brain Aneurysm Foundation website and found clearer definition of a brain aneurysm for you.

> A brain aneurysm, also referred to as a cerebral aneurysm or intracranial aneurysm (IA) is a weak bulging spot on the wall of a brain artery very much like a thin balloon or weak spot on an inner tube. Over time, the blood flow within the artery pounds against the thinned portion of the wall and aneurysms form silently from wear and tear on the arteries. As the artery wall becomes gradually thinner from the dilation, the blood flow causes the weakened wall to swell outward. This pressure may cause the aneurysm to rupture and allow blood to escape into the space around the brain. A ruptured brain aneurysm commonly requires advanced surgical treatment.
>
> http://www.bafound.org/brain-aneurysm-basics
> 5-18-2013

I want to take this time to share some brain aneurysm statistics that I also got from the Brain Aneurysm Foundation's website.

Statistics and Facts

An estimated six million people in the United States have an unruptured brain aneurysm, or 1 in 50 people.

The annual rate of rupture is approximately 8–10 per 100,000 people, or about 30,000 people, in the United States suffer a brain aneurysm rupture. There is a brain aneurysm rupturing every eighteen minutes. Ruptured brain aneurysms are fatal in about 40 percent of cases. Of those who survive, about 66 percent suffer some permanent neurological deficit.

Approximately 15 percent of patients with aneurysmal subarachnoid hemorrhage (SAH) die before reaching the hospital. Most of the deaths from subarachnoid hemorrhage are due to rapid and massive brain injury from the initial bleeding, which is not correctable by medical and surgical interventions.

Four out of 7 people who recover from a ruptured brain aneurysm will have disabilities.

Brain aneurysms are most prevalent in people ages thirty-five to sixty but can occur in children as well. The median age when aneurysmal hemorrhagic stroke occurs is fifty years old, and there are typically no warning signs. Most aneurysms develop after the age of forty.

Most aneurysms are small, about 1/8 inch to nearly one inch, and an estimated 50–80 percent of all aneurysms do not rupture during the course of a person's lifetime. Aneurysms larger than one inch are referred to as giant aneurysms and can pose a particularly high risk and can be difficult to treat.

Women, more than men, suffer from brain aneurysms at a ratio of 3:2.

Ruptured brain aneurysms account for 3–5 percent of all new strokes.

Subarachnoid hemorrhage (SAH) is one of the most feared causes of acute headache upon presentation to the emergency department. Headache accounts for 1–2 percent of the emergency room visits and up to 4 percent of visits to the primary care offices. Among all the patients who present to the emergency room with headaches, approximately 1 percent has subarachnoid hemorrhage. One study put the figure at 4 percent.

Accurate early diagnosis is critical, as the initial hemorrhage may be fatal, may result in devastating neurologic outcomes, or may produce minor symptoms. Despite widespread neuroimaging availability, misdiagnosis or delays in diagnosis occurs in up to 25 percent of patients with subarachnoid hemorrhage (SAH) when initially presenting for medical treatment. Failure to do a scan results in 73 percent

> of these misdiagnoses. This makes SAH a low-frequency, high-risk disease.
>
> There are almost 500,000 deaths worldwide each year caused by brain aneurysms, and half the victims are younger than fifty.
>
> Based on a 2004 study, the combined lost wages of survivors of brain aneurysm rupture and their caretaker for a year were $138,000,000.
>
> The cost of a brain aneurysm treated by clipping via open brain surgery more than doubles in cost after the aneurysm has ruptured. The cost of a brain aneurysm treated by coiling, which is less invasive and is done through a catheter, increases by about 70 percent after the aneurysm has ruptured.
>
> Ten–15 percent of patients diagnosed with a brain aneurysm will harbor more than one aneurysm.
>
> http://www.bafound.org/Statistics_and_Facts
> 5-18-2013

This is the story of when Annie came to visit me. It has taken me almost three years to write this. I found out firsthand that writing a book while recovering from a brain injury was not an easy task. Your deficits can get in the way.

I will discuss the event of Annie's visit itself and the deficits I was left with. I will talk about my recovery and how my life has changed since Annie arrived. You will see that even though I lost significant things due to Annie, I learned to adjust so that I could move forward in my new life. The biggest lesson I learned in my recovery journey was to accept the "new me." I am blessed to be here today and feel honored to be able to share my story with you.

I hope it will help you.

Remembering 2007

I can remember back to one day in December 2007 when I was standing in the living room of the house that Lori, my life partner, and I had purchased some months before. I remember having felt a great sense of accomplishment. It was at that point I found myself reflecting on the fact of how far I had come in my life—from being raised in the foster care system from birth until I chose to go college, then in the '90s being affected by severe depression. The depression was so bad that I was unable to work. I ultimately became homeless for a period of time. I lived out of my car during that time and on friends' couches.

Eventually, I got help for the depression. With the help of Killingsworth, a halfway house for women in Columbia, South Carolina, as well as the South Carolina Vocational Rehabilitation Department and a program called Work in Progress, I was able to get a job and get back on my feet. In 2007, I was standing in a house that we owned. By that point, I had been working as a counselor at Catawba Mental Health for ten years. I was living with someone who loved me and who I loved. On that day, I felt so content and happy. I felt I had overcome so much and finally accomplished my goal of success.

Annie Arrives

February 6, 2008

Little did I know that my life would change on this day. It started out like most any other workday. I was woken up by the alarm clock blaring music from my favorite local radio station. I had to get out of bed and go across the bedroom to turn off the alarm. I learned years ago to put the clock radio across the bedroom. That way I had to get out of bed to turn it off and not just hit the snooze button and roll over back to sleep.

I got ready for work and ate some breakfast. I got in my car and drove to my office which was a thirty-minute drive from our house. I arrived at my office around 8 o'clock, which was about the time I usually arrived at work even though the workday didn't start until 8:30 a.m. I would get there a little early just to have time to settle in for the day.

I went into the building and went to my office. I turned on the computer to check my schedule for the day. I do this each morning so I would know which clients were in my schedule and I could prepare for them. Like if I was to see a child client, I would make sure to pull out some toys I had or paper and crayons. I kept toys, stuffed Garfields, on a bookshelf. Everyone, not just the children, seemed to like my office. Maybe having a large mason jar kept full of chocolate helped!

To be honest, I do not remember most of what happened the day Annie arrived. What I did was interview some of the people who were there to help me put into words the events that make up her arrival.

Ella Franklin, or Ms. Ella as we call her, told me I came to work not feeling well. It had been a long week for us in the office. I did start to see my clients for the day. I apparently did fine until around 2 or 3 p.m. I had a headache, which I thought was just another migraine headache. I had suffered from migraines since I was a young child. I remember being in the front support staff area and telling Ms. Ella I was going to the nurse's office to check my blood pressure, which didn't make sense because I had never had any problems with my blood pressure. I remember being in the nurse's office alone and realizing something was wrong and that I needed to get back to the front office. It is only bits and pieces as to how I got up front but I know I kept praying, asking God to help me. He did! Ella said I got to the front desk window and I told her I needed help. At first she thought I was joking, mostly because I was kind of the office prankster. I did things to help lighten things up around the office. Working in the mental health field can be stressful, so I tried to make my co-workers laugh some.

Ella looked up at me and said my face was beet red. She knew then I was not joking. At some point I got weak, turned a shade of green, and then passed out. She called the emergency code to alert staff that there was a medical emergency in the front office area. I understand all available staff responded, and our psychiatrist and Ms. Ella took the lead in assisting me.

I also interviewed Marissa Wells, my supervisor at the time of this event. I was told that I vomited at times and that at some point I was seizing. Throughout I kept apologizing and kept telling my fellow staff members that I did not want to die. I was apologizing because I knew they had other things to do. I figured I was just sick from a migraine. I hated to be taking up their time. I am very glad Annie arrived while I was at work. They started the steps that saved my life.

Eventually, EMS got to the office and transported me to Chester Regional Medical Center. The ER doctor knew of my migraines because I have had to go to that ER for a shot of medicine for a migraine in the past and this doctor was on duty. He wasn't sure this was a migraine by the way things unfolded, so he ordered a CT scan. Lori was called by Marissa and came to the ER.

The doctor told Lori that he was afraid his hunch was right that I had a hemorrhage on the brain. Since CRMC was not equipped to handle this, he gave Lori two options: I could be airlifted either to Columbia, South Carolina, or to Charlotte, North Carolina. She said Charlotte, so I was airlifted from CRMC Chester, South Carolina, to Carolinas Medical Center in Charlotte, North Carolina. When I was awake and alert, I was told this. I said "I always wanted to ride in a helicopter and now I got to and I don't remember it!" I am told I was in the ICU for four weeks. I had several brain surgeries. One surgery was on February 14, 2008, and I almost didn't make it. They said my vessels fell apart. I suffered a stroke. At some point, I had congested heart failure and had to be put on a respirator.

To give you some more insight on what was happening and the effects on my partner, I got permission from Lori and incorporated e-mails that Lori and her mother sent out to update her family on my condition. I will also comment throughout them to give you a sense of where I was at those points:

> Kelli,
>
> Following you will find many pages of the updates of your health issue of Feb. 2008. I didn't start keeping this report until the week following your first "encounter." You may want to go through it and edit some of the reports. Let me know if I can help with this.
>
> Kathy.

February 16, 2008

Kelli's Report

We just returned from Lori's. Have been down there since Wed. evening. Got home about 1:30 today.

Kelli took a turn for the worse. An angiogram was done Wed. afternoon and two more places showed up; so we went down to be with Lori Wed. night [she was pretty upset and worried]. Then I went with her to the hospital early Thurs. a.m. Kelli went back to surgery after 7:30 a.m. and—boy, oh boy—did they find a mess. Not only were there two more aneurysms, but found a third behind an area where it didn't show up in the angiogram. While the doctor was taking care of the first two, the third "blew" [as he put it] and there was blood all over the place and she lost blood, requiring a transfusion. He had to remove a portion of the right temporal lobe [he said if an area could be removed, it was the right temporal lobe because it wasn't as important for functioning as the rest of the brain. I remember reading about this in my medical records and kind of freaked out! No one told me or I just didn't remember, and reading that a piece of your brain was removed is scary. It reminded me of when we learned of mental patients having lobotomies in the asylums back in the ancient days]. Then he had to do some bypassing and reconstruction work in the problem areas. This man is "the top neurologi-

[illegible] there at Carolinas Medical Center. He told [illegible] he'd done 1500 of these surgeries and had [illegible] lost a one, but Kelli had him worried there for awhile. He said she had "one big Angel sitting on her shoulder" during that surgery [I really believe I have at least one guardian angel. Really, I tell people I have a colony of guardian angels. I figure it is way too much work for one angel to keep me out of harms way. Especially now with my deficits]. He must have spent 15 minutes talking and explaining to us what went on during the surgery and what could be expected afterward. According to him, Kelli had a stroke during all of that, and following the surgery her brain was "in spasms." Said that when something like this happens to the brain, "it gets pissed off" [his words] and goes into these spasms. So, it was almost five hrs. after him talking to us before we were able to see Kelli. She was on a breathing machine and wasn't to be taken off it until sometime today. She had some paralysis in her left hand last night, but was able to grip one's finger this morning when Lori went back in to see her. The doctor can't be sure if and what impairment she may have after all of this, but she will continually be kept in the ICU for another week. I got the impression that rehabilitation will follow later. Lori has already gotten papers filled out and signed [by the surgeon] to be filed with Kelli's insurance company [she has short-term disability insurance] to get her started on disability for the next 3 mos. [that's how long the doctor said she'd have to be out of work]. If there is permanent impairment, she may be out indefinitely. The doctor said he just doesn't know at this point.

Lori is just devastated, won't eat, and is just mentally numb.

Paul stayed at Lori's house yesterday while we were at the hospital, and he put up a new section of their backyard fence to keep their dog in. It was a problem for Lori, because she had to stay outside and watch the dog every time it was let out. Now, she can just let her out and not have to keep an eye on her. Another thing, a lady who worked with Kelli in Chester said she'd be glad to take the dog to her house and look after her while Kelli is confined. So, Lori is going to call the lady and see if she was serious and take her up on that offer. The cats are not a problem, but the dog requires more attention than Lori has time to give and Kelli won't be able to do after she gets out of the hospital.

Paul and I spent all morning this morning cleaning up some of their house.

We are all just worried and numb from all of this and are especially concerned about what this is all doing to Lori. I'm just hoping she can hold up. She is already starting to worry about their finances now that Kelli is going to be out of work for so long. But we told her to just take it all one step at a time. She breaks down and cries at the least little thing. I had to console her three times while we were at the hospital after the doctor talked with us. She has had to miss a lot of her own work, but fortunately her bosses are good in "working with her." One of the bosses has a doctor wife and she even called at the hospital to check on things and told Lori that Kelli's surgeon is "the best." They have even offered to let Lori sleep over at their house when she needs to so she won't have to be driving back and forth from Rock Hill to Charlotte. They are very nice to her.

Feb. 19, 2008

We just returned this afternoon from a two-night stay with Lori—she was pretty upset Sat. night about how Kelli is doing. Saturday, Kelli wasn't responding to commands and wasn't responding to Lori speaking to her. So we felt that Lori needed to have someone at home with her for a few days—thus, we went back to be with her.

We went to the hospital yesterday a.m. to visit Kelli and she was sedated and sleeping most of the time. However, when Lori spoke to her and told her that we were there, she responded with "that's good." Before we got there, she was awake enough to ask Lori how her little dog was doing, so that was a bit encouraging. But she was running a fever yesterday and was being given medication for that. She was scheduled to have another angiogram this morning but that was put off for awhile because she's had so much radiation and already had 3 previous angiograms. She still doesn't move her left leg, but does move the left arm a bit. But she doesn't grip one's finger when asked to. [Let me tell you, the doctors asked me to squeeze their pointer fingers so often that I would dream about it! I dreamt once I was sleeping in my mom's bed in Connecticut. She was sleeping in her spare bedroom. The doctors were coming up to the bed and telling me to squeeze their finger. They kept coming over and over. I told them they were gonna wake my mother if they didn't stop. Boy, the medication they had me on sure had my mind working. I had other crazy dreams during my stay at CMC]. This is going to be a long recovery period; so I'll not report much for awhile unless it is of extreme importance.

Thanks for your concern and prayers.

Kathy

February 20, 2008

How is Kelli doing today? Hopefully she'll show some improvement. Well, let us know tonight how Kelli is doing.

We love you,
Mom

Friday's report (2-22-08) From Lori

I ran into Dr. Van Der Veer yesterday morning as I was going in and he said her BP dropped too low for them and she went lethargic, so they changed up her drips or whatever and got it back to the level that it needed to be. He seemed very hopeful and said he wasn't interested in doing an angiogram because it would only be for "looking around just to be looking around" right now. After talking with him, I went in and saw her being fed breakfast and her eyes were brighter. However, when she went to sleep, she went into a strange dream stage. Yesterday afternoon, she had heartburn and belly cramps that was making her really uncomfortable. And I think that belly pain was making her breathing labored. She wasn't babbling the crazy talk, but she is having some crazy dreams apparently.

Sent: Friday, February 22, 2008, 2:01 p.m. (from Lori)

Subject: rough morning

We had to put Kelli on a ventilator this morning. Yesterday when her BP dropped, they pumped her with tons of fluids. Now she has too much fluid around her heart and in the right lung. When I got in this morning, she was on an IPAP that was forcing air into her and she was breathing like she was in a marathon. It was upsetting for me and the nurse to watch so she called the medical doc [Dr. Hudson] and he talked to both of us and said that they can keep her sedated and on a vent for a couple of days so they can clear up the fluid in her chest. This way she won't suffer and she won't remember any of it. [Thank goodness I don't remember any of this. It scares me each time I read it! To be on a ventilator and having the episode I had with the breathing.] Whew, that was rough to take. I'm good now that she is resting and on the vent. I called Marge and let her know. She is going to fly down sometime next week. They are getting a bunch of snow right now. Marge is my biological mother. She lives in West Hartford, Connecticut. I met her for the first time when I was in tenth grade. Many people say I look a lot like her.

Monday, Feb. 25, 2008—Update from Lori

The nurse said this morning that Kelli looks to be improving. Dr. Adamson is pleased that her left arm is moving and she is gripping some with the left hand. He didn't think she would be able to do that much. [I still remember focusing on the need to squeeze my left hand. I heard the doctor saying something about not regaining movement in my left arm/hand. I kept thinking to myself to squeeze or move it while I was laying there. There was a co-worker at my office who had a stiff left arm as a result of a brain injury. She does very well with it and I always admired her, but I remembered that and didn't want a stiff arm. I know my focusing like that made a difference] So the nurse said that it is looking rehab-able. Dr. Hudson wants to leave her on the vent for a couple more days at least and the white blood count is coming down. They are bringing down her BP also, so the nurse feels that the spasms are letting up also. She needs to do a bowel movement and they are giving her all sorts of things to get that to happen. I'll bet she feel SO MUCH better when that happens.

Tues. Feb. 26, 2008—Update from Lori

Kelli is still improving, but still sedated and on the respirator. They have taken her off the Mannitol [for brain swelling]. Her Doppler numbers are still coming down and her intracranial pressure [ICP] is also coming down. They also raised her drain line. Don't know if they are doing a chest x-ray today or tomorrow to see how the pneumonia is clearing. I think she is alternating movement of her left arm and leg. Today she moves the left leg ever so slightly, but not the left arm. The nurse brought her awake for a little while I was in there this morning and I talked to her, but it is hard to tell if she is focused enough to listen.

More news later,

Wed., Feb. 27, '08—Update from Lori

Still on respirator, but nurse says her chest is a lot clearer today. When I left at 11:00 a.m. nurse was waiting on call back from doctor re: raising BP because the Doppler test numbers had gone up today. In some respects the doctors don't think the Doppler is accurate and since her ICP is low and other responses are good, they may ignore it somewhat. I will find out this afternoon what they want to do about the Doppler numbers. Today marks 3 weeks in ICU.

Reports from Lori

Thurs., Feb. 28, '08—Update

Another day of good news. When I got to her room this morning, Kelli had her eyes open, but still a bit groggy. When I left, they said they should have her off the vent by the time I go back this afternoon. Dr. Adamson came in the room while I was there and said to me that she has "turned the corner." He said that she should not have any bad surprises now and the next steps are rehabbing. He said it is possible for her to get to a regular room next week. The nurse said she has to be breathing well enough on her own and off the Dopamine before they release her from ICU.

Fri., Feb. 29, '08—Update

Kelli is off the respirator, but still on the feeding tube and oxygen mask (and has a sore throat). She's not talking, but is awake. I don't know about reporting all of this, because I think she has come out of this with some depression. She is not the same Kelli I know. The nurse says this is normal behavior and I'm sure she has weird feelings after being out of it for a week. She has an "I don't care" type of affect. I hope it's not hopelessness. I told her that the doctors are pleased with her progress and that she is doing really good. At least she nodded when I said that we will take this one step at a time because she can rehab and get back to normal ["Back to normal." Lori and I both wanted that! Annie changed mine and Lori's life as you will see later. Both of us did want me to be back to normal, and then our lives could go back to normal. I couldn't see how I was going to be normal after Annie visited me. One thing I do remember about this time that probably played into my attitude was the weird feeling in my head. I kept thinking, "This must have been what people felt like that were scalped by the Indians in the pioneer days." It was like my scalp felt separated from my head, that they had peeled it back and then laid it back on top of my head. I wondered if my hair was going to be affected. One thing I have always liked about my looks was my hair! Annie has helped me to not only like my hair, but to appreciate it. I have thick, healthy hair. This helps to cover all the scars]. I just worry about severe depression.

What really bothered me is that I had mentioned to her after the 1st surgery that we could get the Wii game for her when she gets home and she was excited about it. But today, when I mentioned it, she shook her head like she didn't want it and why bother. I know I have to keep talking to her about looking forward to getting out of the hospital and going home and some fun things she likes to do. It's early and she's not even out of ICU, so she will come around when she gets off the medicine and feels better.

Mon., Mar. 3, '08—Update

Kelli is still on the feeding tube this morning, but she is hungry and thirsty. They are still waiting on the speech therapist to do a swallowing test to make sure she can eat and drink on her own. Poor thing wants some food now! I hope by the time I go back this afternoon, they will have tested her.

Dr. Adamson came by and told the nurse that the Doppler numbers are good and down and they are weaning her off the Dopamine. We may get her in a regular room tomorrow. Cross your fingers.

Tues., Mar, 4, '08 (a.m.)

When I got back to the hospital yesterday afternoon, the nurse said she was having trouble swallowing and the speech therapist said they would wait a couple more days to see how she does. So, she is still on the feeding tube. I'll see what the doctor, etc. says today. So, she may be in ICU at least a couple more days. Poor thing is hungry and thirsty and can't swallow yet. Apparently the muscles get weak while the tube is down the throat. I talked to a lady at bowling last night who said her mother, at age 56, had surgery for her bleeding aneurysm and after a month of rehab, she was able to leave the hospital. She said her mother has some memory problems, but was doing fine otherwise. Her mother is in her 60s now. So, it sounds like she can rehab out of this, but I can't know how much she can do after that. By the way, I found that Kelli has a supplemental disability policy that will send claim forms to me. It was another deduction from her paycheck and I called about it and learned that it is another disability policy. How 'bout that?

Tues., (p.m.)

Well even though Kelli is still not swallowing, they have transfer orders to move her to regular room if one comes open this afternoon. They have scheduled a swallow test tomorrow—one w/ dye and x-ray to see what's going on. So I hope she can at least move to another room today or tomorrow. Tell everyone thank you for their thoughts and concern for us. It means a lot.

Thurs., Mar. 6, '08—Update

Kelli now in a room—

I had a rough time last night. Kelli scooches all over the bed and always ends up sideways in the bed and leg(s) hanging off. I'm allowed to use the cell phone, so I called Donna and I was no more than a minute on the phone when in the corner of my eye I see Kelli handing me something and saying "throw this away." She had pulled her feeding tube almost all the way out! [I remember this!] I called the nurse and she came in and began shoving it back down her nose. Made Kelli gag and squirm. The night shift nurse came by and put in another tube and tortured Kelli all over again. The first nurse had tied

Kelli's right arm down so she wouldn't pull the tube again, but the night nurse said she didn't believe in tying the patients down. I swear if I find out that she pulled the tube out last night after I left, I will give some ultimatums. She does not know what she is pulling or what she's doing.

The reason she was still on the feeding tube is because she didn't do well on the barium swallow test. And, I think she didn't do well is because the nurse said when they took her, she was more than half asleep. I'm sure I can't swallow when I'm asleep either!

They said the therapists had her sitting in a chair yesterday afternoon, so they are already starting to work with her. She wiggled her left toes last night. She still can't follow fingers with her eyes going to the left yet.

On top of that, Marge called me while I was in the room and I let her talk w/ Kelli. But she kept saying I should do this and do that and call the doctor about every little thing. When I told her about Kelli pulling the feeding tube, she didn't realize that the tube goes through the nose and down to the stomach. She thought it was a tube straight through the belly to the stomach. I had to explain. I was already frustrated and I didn't need someone to tell me what to do. I've been in that hospital 2x a day for a month now. And Sussana, coworker of Lori's, here at the office tells me to be patient and not to push to get Kelli out of ICU. Whatever.

Later. [Lori was wonderful throughout all this. I did not feel pressured by her to get out of the hospital. She challenged me when I needed it. I did things to help also. For example, since I had left side neglect syndrome, my brain wasn't recognizing the left very well. I got where I was listening to Beyonce's song, "Irreplaceable," just to keep playing the "To the left, to the left" over and over, trying to program my brain. This was just one thing I could do to work on this deficit, because when they would put my meal tray in front of me, I would miss items on it, only because I did not look to the left on the tray. It was such a task to learn, but my brain eventually did it!]

Friday, 3/7/08

Kelli was determined that she needed to go to the Verizon store last night. She wants me to give her cell phone to her. I let her hold it yesterday, but she held it upside down and just looked at it. She's so funny. [So glad I provided some humor in all this madness. I continue to keep some humor and positivity as part of my recovery process.] She squirms in the bed, but it wasn't as bad as the day before. The night nurse told me last night that the night before, she found Kelli about completely sideways in the bed, with her head hanging out one side and her feet the other side! Now that's she's more alert, she wants me there longer and I just don't have the time on a weekday. I didn't get home 'till after 9:00 because I needed to go to the store and get gas. And went another night that I couldn't do the laundry. Ugh.

Message 2—

If I do some laundry at the house in the morning I'll probably get up there by 12:30 or 1:00.

I got a call about 20 minutes ago from rehab representative of some kind at the hospital who said that I will get a call Monday from Dr. Shannon, rehab doctor, about a "plan of care." They may be transferring her to an acute rehab place by Tuesday or Wednesday. Apparently they want to know how much training I can undergo as her home caregiver. So I will have a lot of questions next week.

Mon., Mar., 10, '08—Update

Kelli passed her swallow test today, but can only ingest puree food and thickened liquids. [Let me tell you, that was horrible! I hated the texture of the thickening mixture. I was really wanting a juicy cheeseburger!] I have not heard from the rehab doctor yet and she had not come by while I was there at lunchtime. I suppose we are headed in the right direction, but inch by inch.

Tues., Mar., 11, '08

I have yet to hear from this "Dr. Shannon." Marge is flying in the afternoon. They removed the feeding tube yesterday, because she had passed the swallow test. They give her thick fluids and puree food for now. Kelli is probably looking for me now. I bowled last night and didn't see her last night. I'll go over in a little bit. And then Marge will come in this afternoon…

Wed., Mar. 12

It has been a crazy day. I've talked w/ both a CMC social worker and case manager from BCBS. She is not getting enough PT in the regular room that will meet the criteria to get into "acute" rehab, so we need to get her into a "sub-acute" facility which will be a skilled nursing home situation. Her ins [insurance] will only pay 20 days [$6000] for a place in SC, so we are looking at some places in Rock Hill for transfer. I was assured that she will get serious PT so that she can be somewhat mobile to meet criteria for acute rehab [Carolinas Rehab, etc.]. The BCBS case manager sounds like she will be a big help for me in holding my hand through this in looking at therapy notes and doctor records, etc. On top of all of that, yes, Marge got in last a night and stayed with me at the house. She called me from the hospital this morning to say that while she went to get a newspaper and the nurses were changing the bed while Kelli was in a chair, they left her in the chair on a bedpan alone. Kelli always squirms while on the bedpan and leaned forward too far and fell in the floor. [Now what really happened is I was left sitting in a chair on a bedpan. I was done. I then decided I could get myself back in bed. I didn't see the need to wait for the nurse. Part of a brain injury is not recognizing your deficits. At that point, I was not able to totally recognize all my deficits. When the nurses came back in, they found me on the floor twirling in a circle! This was because only my right arm and leg were moving. Yet in my mind I was trying to stand up! This is also why I would end up sideways in the bed. I would think I was moving myself but only my right arm and leg were actually moving. I still giggle a little bit when I think about this. Can you imagine being one of those nurses, walking into my room and seeing a grown women twirling on the floor! It's okay! You can laugh. I did.] We hope her head is OK, but they did a CT scan to be sure. Don't know if the results are back on that yet.

[I did hit my head, but there was no damage. Maybe, by that point, my brain was really tough as nails!]

What else could go crazy?

Thurs. Mar 13

BCBS is Blue Cross Blue Shield and her benefit for this skilled nursing home is only $6000 for 20 days. Got to see Dr. Hudson this morning and he didn't know about the fall, but we talked about the rehab. He said that she may not meet criteria yet to be able to do 3 hours of rehab and needs to work her way up to that. I don't think she is getting much in the regular room. The BCBS SC state plan will only pay for the 20 days in South Carolina, so that is why we have to look in Rock Hill. I am going down there today to visit a couple of the places that BCBS will pay for in RH.

Marge flew out this morning. She is fine accept [except] for telling me I need to do this and I need to tell so and so about this and make sure to report and demand this and blah, blah, blah. Other than that she's great. They didn't call her "Sarge Marge" for nothing'when she worked for the State of Conn. [Yep, my mom can be tough but I think Annie visiting me might have scared her a bit and that was her way of trying to be helpful. I would think it would be hard on a parent if something happened to their child like a visit from Annie. They would probably feel helpless because they have no control over the outcome, so I know mom might have been sharp with Lori but I guess I can understand where she was coming from. I'm just glad they worked it out.]

Thurs. afternoon, Mar 13, '08

Went back to Rock Hill to visit RH Rehab and the Agape places. At RH Rehab I got a tour by the social worker and got to sit and talk w/ the Physical Therapist. At Agape I toured with a couple needing to put his mother in and the rooms were really nice, but they would not let me talk to a therapist or really inspect the therapy room [because I don't think they had much of one]. I asked two more times about talking to the therapist at Agape and when she said no, I said I'll go now, how do I get out of here? I'll try to call you later tonight.

Fri. afternoon, Mar. 14, '08

I got to see the PA and Dr. Adamson while I was in at lunch-time. They both said that they are consulting a pediatric neurosurgeon [Dr. McLanahan] because he is the expert on shunts. They said the ventricles in the brain look enlarged, which may mean fluid in there and may be causing her headaches. So, we need to wait and see what Dr. McLanahan wants to do. Otherwise she is doing OK. She's being a wuss and not sitting in the chair more than 30 minutes. She started wussin' out at 10 minutes and I kept fussing at her to avoid calling the nurse. She made it for a half hour. [Sometime after McLanahan saw me, it was decided that a shunt was needed to help remove the excess fluid out of the ventricles.]

Wed. Mar. 19, '08

She is doing well, except for soreness from the surgery. She has an incision behind her right ear and on her stomach area and they are sore. She will have another barium swallow test today and hopefully get the green light to drink regular liquids and maybe better food. Now, she can hardly get a pill down with the thick liquid. Other than the soreness, she has no setbacks from this shunt surgery. She had the same anesthetist as the second surgery. You might remember him with the accent. He is very nice. The surgeon looked like an old farmer in scrubs. They are still getting her up and she is off the catheter. BUT, last night we put her on the potty chair and she was so happy to pee regularly in the pot, however, she wasn't scotched back enough and half of her pee went in the floor. She had no idea that was happening. I got towels to soak up what I could see on the floor, but saw that it flowed under the bed! I was so tired I had to leave at 7:00 and no one had come up yet with a mop. When I go at lunch it had better not smell of urine or I will [be] getting' on somebody. Because I don't think anyone has mopped the floor since she's been in there. I would have done it myself if there was a mop and bucket to be found on the floor.

And so it goes.

Wed. afternoon—3/19/08

The medical and neuron docs have to discharge her medically, but her foster mom, Judith, came up today and just called me before leaving and said that Kelli walked to the door [with the PT] and back to the bed. [Learning to walk again was not an easy task but I was determined. I kept making it into little challenges. I was walking with assistance at this point, then I graduated to using a walker, then to a cane, and finally, after two years from the arrival of Annie, I was walking on my own without any aids.] If she keeps that up, I have to think she can go straight to acute rehab when she is medically able.

Thurs. Mar. 20

Well Kelli would have been moved down to Rock Hill today except she has a bad headache and got nauseated when they got her up. She is having another CT scan today and Dr. McLanahan will take a look at things to see if she needs any adjustment w/ that shunt. She walked/shuffled w/ walker and therapists today out and into the hallway, sat down for a short rest and walked back to the bed. She is making good progress for sure. She said the headaches are really bad though. So I might get her into the sub-acute rehab soon

Mon. Mar. 24, '08

I talked by Kelli's cell phone with Dr. McLanahan's nurse practitioner this morning and then later this morning they did a needle thing in the back of her head to check the pressure with the shunt. Kelli called me crying saying the procedure was really painful. [I did cry like a baby and I think I pissed the doctor off because I was moving my head. It was painful but I was being a wuss, I think because I had been through so much already. Since then, I have had my shunt tapped and have done just fine.] Both I and Kelli told Julie that her headaches have been debilitating since the shunt was put in. So we wait to see what the pressure situation is and then…I don't know what. They were bringing her pain medicine, but I need to talk with someone about better pain medicine. That Lortab only takes the edge off.

Tues., Mar. 25, '08

Just got a call from a girl from Carolinas Institute of Rehab [CIR] who said that she has been looking at Kelli's situation and that once this shunt situation is fixed, they can take her straight into acute rehab. So, I don't have to send her to Rock Hill first. Yay! I saw Dr. McLanahan early this a.m. and he said he wants to tap into her shunt again (we will need to sedate her somehow) so he can get more info on it and then decide whether he needs to go back in and put in a programmable shunt or not. He said that it is possible that the shunt is draining the fluid too well or she doesn't need it because the CT scan looks OK. So, I don't know what will transpire tomorrow. But at least, I know that when we take care of the headaches and shunt, she can go straight to CIR.

Tues. afternoon

They will do whatever rehab she needs at CIR and then send her home. However, they want to know what the home situation is before sending her home. She will need someone with her 24/7 when she gets home. I have already talked with Kathy Wilds about getting some folks who can help and hopefully Marge, Judith, and Donna can come and stay ONE AT A TIME. Now that I've talked with Leslie at CIR, I feel better. She said they are ready for her and have a call into BCBS, which I know will approve. CIR is "in-network" and has no limit to her stay.

Wed. p.m. 3/26/08

Early this morning, Dr McLanahan tried to do another tap into her head w/ dye and go under the scan, but she was too fearful, so he scheduled to do it under some anesthesia mid-day. I went again at noon and went down w/ her and left her in their hands. He wants to send the dye through the shunt and see how it is really working. I'll go back after work and see if there are any news/results of this testing.

Update–Mar. 27, '08

Dr. McLanahan said this morning that the flow with the shunt was working fine although it is still possible that it works too well. They found no infection but he wants to study the fluid more. He wants to keep her on the floor and see how she does today and tomorrow with sitting up and some walking and if she is still having problems, he said he could do something "this weekend." I don't know what that means. I've sent a request for the records from the neurologist in Rock Hill for records about her neck problems and take them to CMC and let them know about that problem in case it has any bearing.

Thurs. afternoon—

Kelli called me this afternoon and said the nurse told her she is scheduled for a procedure tomorrow, but not sure what McLanahan is doing, but that he or his assistant will talk to her about it. I'll bet he wants to change out the shunt. I hope to learn more when I go over after work. She probably needs a shunt that is more adjustable. [They did put in a programmable shunt and it is something out of Star Trek. When I have to have it adjusted, the doctor plugs into a computer what level they want the shunt set on, then they take a wand that is connected to the computer and hold it over my head at the area where the shunt is. The wand communicates the information to the shunt. How cool is that!]

Lori called to let us know that Kelli is being moved from the hospital to the rehab facility next door this afternoon—just one day short of being in the hospital 8 wks. Hope to see a lot of improvement in her recovery now.

Thurs. Apr. 3, '08

Yes, she was moved yesterday afternoon and they put her in with an older lady. Don't know the story about the infection isolation. Kelli was weepy last night before I left. It reminded me when I started at Carolina. She just wants to go home and [it] is hard for her to understand that she is just not able to go home even for a quick visit. It was hard to leave her, but I think she went to sleep soon after that, according the roommate (Ms. Tucker). [Boy, it was tough that night. I wanted to go home. I was tired of hospitals.] I got over there this morning and the occupational therapist helped her take a shower, which made her tired and she weeped [wept] a bit because of that. I told her she is doing better than most and that she will work up to better stamina. [I didn't believe that! I really felt like I was spent and was never gonna get better, yet there was the survivor deep inside me that would not let me give up!]

Mon. Apr. 7, '08

The rehab social worker called and said the "team" will be ready to discharge her to home on Friday. Yes, Friday, April 11. However, the health ins case worker said if I do not have people to be with her round the clock, we cannot send her home. Oh boy.

Waking up

I don't remember any of this. First thing I remember is waking up in a hospital room with Lori and her parents talking with some nurse or doctor. They were talking about me having brain damage and not being sure how bad it was. They talked about how my left side was going to be affected and it could be that I would not be able to use my left side. I thought to myself that I had to do whatever it takes to make my arms and legs work. I began at that moment taking my left hand and concentrating on squeezing a soft pillow I had laying under the left hand. I would lay there squeezing the pillow, determined I would use the left hand. I remember the first time I opened a can of soda with my left hand, people were impressed. Waking up after having Annie visit me and then having brain surgery, I felt pretty foggy. I kept thinking it was the medication they had me on. In time, I came to understand that my brain had gone through so much with Annie's visit and all. It was weak and would need time to heal.

I remained in the hospital for a total of about ten weeks. I was depressed, missing being at home. I missed my dog Kaci. At some point, Kaci was brought to rehab to visit. I was in a wheelchair, but that did not stop her from being excited to see me. She jumped right up into my lap! It felt good to see her.

Just like my will to survive kicked in and helped keep me alive when Annie first showed up, that will to survive also played a big part in my rehab. I would get frustrated with a task or with my progress but I wouldn't give up. I knew I had to keep trying.

Going Home

Finally, I was well enough to go home. I was so ready to go home, but I didn't quite grasp yet that this was only the beginning of my recovery. I wanted to be back to "normal" and get back to my life.

My first day home was strange. I didn't recognize our house when Lori pulled into the driveway. We went in the house and I had to reacquaint myself with our home. It did come back. Having Kaci jumping for joy that I was home helped. Starting that first day, I had the feeling that I was living in someone else's life.

I had to go to outpatient rehabilitation. There was one in Rock Hill, South Carolina where I lived. I went to Health South Rehabilitation for physical therapy, occupational therapy, and speech therapy. The staff was the best and worked hard to help me get better.

In speech therapy, I learned skills to help with my memory along with other skills. I had a hard time at first understanding that there was so much more to speech therapy than working on one's speech. I finally was able to wrap my brain around the concept. I had a lot of homework assignments in speech therapy but it sure was worth it! In occupational therapy, they had me do a variety of things! I was given some clay that was in a small container with a lid. It was bright pink. My first thought was it was Play-Doh! I loved plying with Play-Doh and Silly Putty growing up. They had me use it at different times. Rolling it, needing [kneading] it, etc. The first time I pulled some out, I learned it was not anything like Play-Doh. This clay was made of a thicker consistency. I figured out that by working with this clay, it was working the muscles in my hands and arms. They also had me doing fun activities that I knew were to help with some things I was unaware of. One day, I made cupcakes as part of my OT. They kept treatment interesting and I was seeing it helping me.

I had the best physical therapist. Her name was Alexa White. She was very encouraging, yet pushed me to do my best. She helped me in so many ways. Due to the events in my childhood, it had always been hard for me to trust people, and yet her personality was such that it was easy for me to trust her. I even told her about my life story. By trusting her, it made it easier to follow anything she had me do. This was important since part of what we worked on in PT was balance! One exercise I had to do was Alexa would have me stand on a board that had a curve on the bottom of it. I would then have to learn to balance myself on the board without falling. Alexa was so great at encouraging me to take on this task. I was nervous, yet I knew with her help, I could achieve the goal! She had me start out in between the parallel bars. That way I could grab on to them if I needed to. I remember working on that task for so long. I'd get frustrated! I sometimes would start thinking, "I will never be able to do this!" Then I would stop myself from that thought process. I began to tell myself that I can do this! Eventually, I was able to balance myself on the board!

I was so excited to see how my therapies were helping my recovery. I made sure to keep all my appointments at Health South. It was within walking distance from my house. Yes, with my cane, I would walk to treatment! I figured even though it tired me out sometimes, it was good exercise. I hope I just gave you some inspiration to go to any lengths to get what you need. I was determined to get better. Cab fare was way too much and I couldn't work out getting a ride. This was what I had to do until I was cleared to drive.

Along with getting my treatment at Health South, I had other doctors helping me. For example, I had an eye specialist to help with my vision deficits. You see, the stroke caused damage to my optic nerve which is causing the blind spot in my left peripheral vision. The first doctor we went to for consultation about this told me there was no surgery to fix it and basically to accept it as is. Well, that did not go over well with me! I was eventually referred to an eye specialist Dr. Gina Beasley who specialized in visual deficits due to brain injuries. At my first appointment, they tested me to really see how my eyes were doing. The test also showed how much field of vision I had.

The most amazing thing was when the doctor showed me how they could move my blind spot over! She had me look in the lens that they used to test what lens you needed. It was through that where she showed me that with prisms in my lens, it would move the blind spot over enough out of my field of vision. It was so nice to walk and not worry about bumping into things. This also helped make it better for me to be able to drive.

Driving

I had not driven a car since the day Annie arrived. I was informed by my physiatrist that I could not drive until I went through a driving evaluation and he wrote a letter clearing me to drive again.

Now, before I go any further, I'm sure you may be wondering—as I did the first time I heard the name—what is a *physiatrist*? My understanding is that a physiatrist is a medical doctor who specialized in rehabilitation medicine. Someone told me that he was the conductor in the orchestra of my recovery services. I was fortunate to have the best physiatrist a person could have in our area, Dr. W. His only downfall was that he was a Steelers fan. I always made sure to wear my Carolina Panthers colors when I had an appointment with him. We gave each other a hard time. He told me one time that I was progressing very well, except that his hope for my full recovery is that I'll be a Steelers' fan. We laughed and I assured him that Annie did not affect my loyalty for my Carolina Panthers!

Dr. W worked hard with me to get me on the right medications to help my brain in its recovery. There was a point when I had a seizure and it was Dr. W's job to figure out what medication to put me on to help me not have more seizures. He was helping me with medications for alertness but had to be sure not to give too much that it would cause another seizure. He worked hard and finally got me on the right combination of medications that helped keep my brain alert when it needed to be but prevented any further seizures.

Now, back to the driving evaluation. Lori drove me to the Carolinas Rehab where I had the appointment for the evaluation. I couldn't figure out how they were going to evaluate my driving there. Once we arrived, the evaluator greeted us and had me fill out a questionnaire related to my injury and my abilities at that time—questions about memory, etc. After finishing the questionnaire, the evaluator interviewed me, then she escorted me to a room where she said they would be testing my reflexes. Basically, they were testing that I could react quickly enough for driving.

They had a machine/computer in this room that had two pedals on it just like in a car. As I sat, my feet could touch the pedals. In front of me was a box that had three lights on it. I was instructed to touch the brake if the red light came on. Boy, this was a lot harder than you might think! I somehow passed though. After the testing and interview, the evaluator had one recommendation—that I have a GPS to help me get from one location to another. It was funny because I had wanted a GPS long before Annie arrived but Lori wasn't too keen on the idea. Now, this lady was recommending I get one to help me with driving. She explained to Lori that people with memory issues have benefited from using GPS to keep track of where they were going. I named my GPS *Sophia*, after the character on the "Golden Girls." She was so good at telling stories to give advice to the other girls.

I was then told that this was only the first step in getting my driving privileges back. For the next step, I had to make an appointment with a driving school and pass their evaluation. We were given the number of a driving school to contact to set up the next step.

The driving school was located out of Charlotte, North Carolina. Lori called and made arrangements for us to meet the instructor at Lori's office parking lot. This was on Moorhead Street in Charlotte. Lori drove and I was nervous thinking about being tested behind the wheel. Other than practicing the last couple weeks on my street for about a block with Lori in the car, I had not driven a car since Annie arrived. When the instructor arrived, I was told I will be driving their car. Yes! It had "Student Driver" on it. Now, I was going to get in a strange car and have to drive around Charlotte! I was nervous but I was determined. I wanted my independence and I knew I needed to drive to have that. The instructor had me get in the driver seat of the car and she got in the passenger seat. She would tell me where she wanted me to drive. I did my best to follow her directions. I felt like I was back in high school doing my driver's test!

I was nervous also because I had the blindness on my left peripheral vision. They did fit me with glasses that had prisms in the lens that moved the blind spot over to give me a wider field of vision. I guess I wasn't 100 percent confident on that day and worried I might mess up while I was being tested. I drove through the city very well, keeping my speed at the appropriate limits and staying alert the entire time. The instructor wrote up her report which passed me. She said I had to give it to my physiatrist for him to write the letter clearing me to drive.

It was another two weeks before I saw the physiatrist but he wrote the letter! For the first two weeks, I had to have someone in the car with me. Boy, Lori hated that. I guess I scared her when I drove. After that, I was on my own with Sophia!

Driving is such a privilege! I do not take it for granted at all. For me to drive, I have to talk to myself. Sounds crazy, I know, but it's true. I have to tell my brain what to do. It's not second nature anymore. From the time I start the car I start reminding my brain to "focus." I will say to myself, "Focus," or "Alert in your lane," pretty much my entire trip. I have found it helps to keep me focused on the driving to stop my brain from thinking of other things. If I don't repeat those statements, I'm afraid I would day dream and that wouldn't be good. Driving used to be relaxing for me; not so much now. Still, I am so very thankful to be able to drive.

To be honest, I believe the reason I am able to drive is because the Lord has been with me and guided me. I believe I have guardian angels helping me out. I wish I could recall specific times for you but there have been times that I recall saying, "I know I only got through that untouched because of my angels." Needless to say, with the help of my guardian angels and Sophia, I have been driving and I'm glad that is one thing that Annie did not take away from me! I don't want you to think by what I just said that I'm unsafe to drive—I am a very safe driver. I just know I am blessed to be able to drive after having Annie come visit me. I explain to people I can't just run out and meet you at the new pub, for example. I have to have an address to put into Sophia so that she can guide me to the location. Yes, this can be frustrating, especially when someone assumes I know the area and says things like, "You know, the road across from the Bi-Lo, then turn left." Okay! No, I do not know and I will not remember what you just said. I have to focus on driving when I'm behind the wheel. Using Sophia helps me to do just that! Remember, it is perfectly normal to use any gadget (GPS, iPad, etc.) that will assist you in your pursuit to live an independent life.

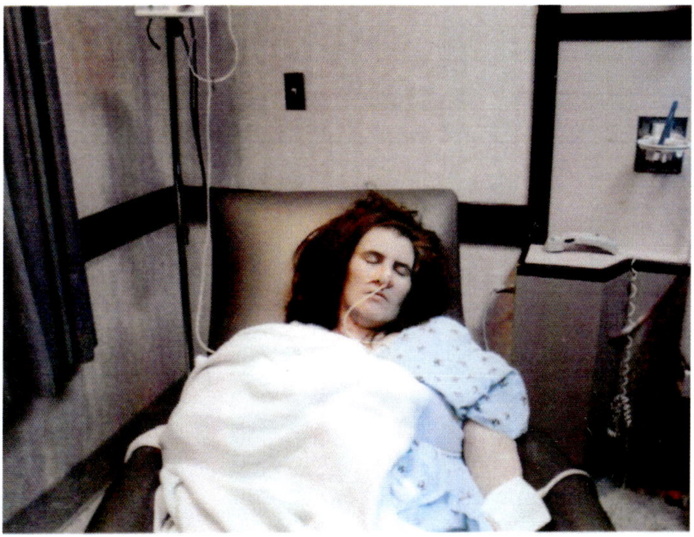

2008 with feeding tube.

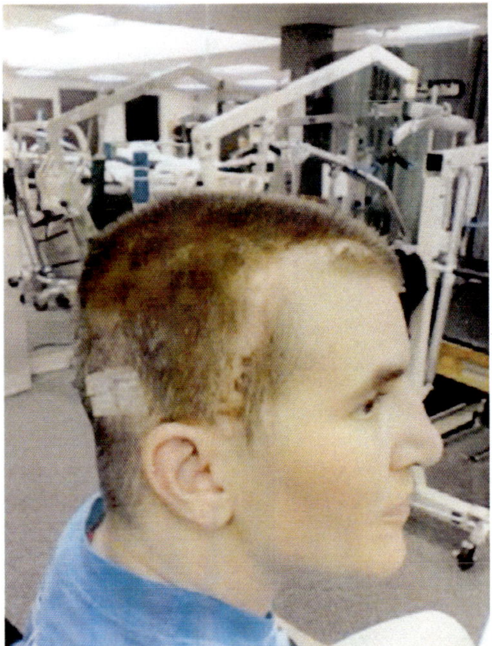

2008 after long hair was shaved off.

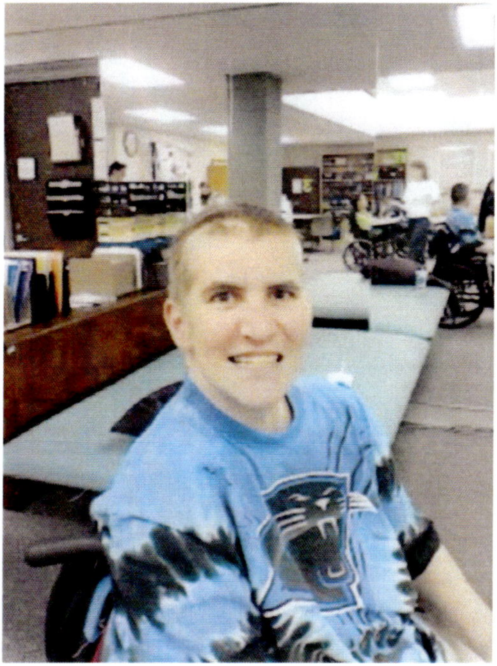

2008 after long hair was shaved off.

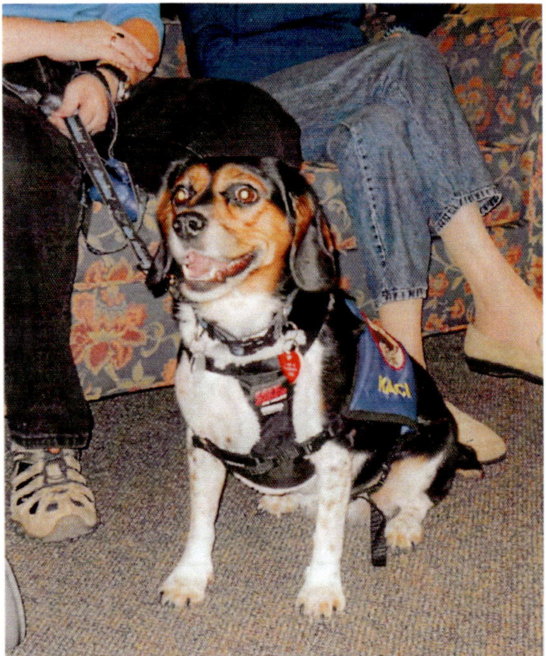

Kaci on a pet therapy visit

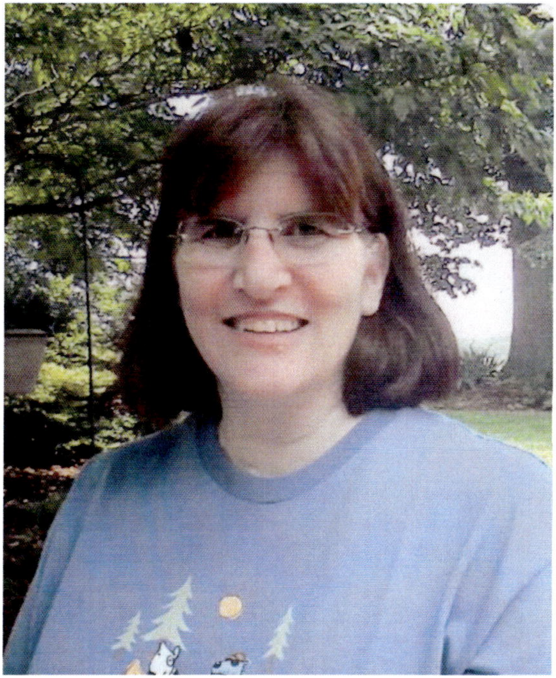

2011

Motivations

Along with attending rehab, I looked to find things I could do to help me with my recovery. I resumed watching the *Golden Girls* and the *Ellen DeGeneres Show*, both of which helped me laugh. Laughter is good for you. When I watched these shows and laughed, I would almost forget I was recovering from a brain injury. The same thing was true when I would sit down to watch my Carolina Panthers play. I have been a Panthers' fan from day one but I never thought they would influence my recovery the way they did. I think it was 2008, but I don't recall the exact game. I was in the hospital, and the game was on TV in my room. The score at halftime was visitors 17, Panthers 0. I remember others in the room being upset with the Panthers once again. I just kept staring at the TV. What I saw was the players huddled together. Our players came together and the camera showed them coming in and I could see the fight in their eyes. They were not giving up! They were fighting to the end! By the way, we won that game! That inspired me—no matter how bad this recovery journey gets, I cannot give up. I say, "The Panthers don't give up, neither do I!" I even took various Panther stickers and decorated my cane with them. I figured if I had to use a cane, why not have some fun and represent my team? I watch every game, cheering them from my living room. It is therapeutic as well as fun. I am a forever Panther fan!

Blogs

I went online and found that the *Ellen DeGeneres Show* had an online community. I joined and had a web page on there. I began blogging my recovery on my web page. These are those blogs:

New Blogger

I am new at blogging and due to an aneurysm rupturing and hemorrhaged in my brain in Feb. 2008, typing is not as simple as it was before. My brain doesn't recognize my left side. I am going to copy and paste something I wrote the other day to help people understand the effects of the aneurysm.

Added by Kelli Schoen
on September 15, 2008 at 7:28pm—

Just Another Day

I slept some. I finally figured out how to add photos on my page. Yeah. I don't feel as bad as the last couple days, but still trying to get even better. I hope you all enjoy the photos. One dog and four cats make life interesting.

My first full day at home I slept most of it. I am somewhat woozy, hope it is just the after affects from the surgery. I want so bad to wake up one day and not be woozy, lightheaded, sick to my stomach, or have a headache. This being sick is for the birds. I want to get up and be productive. The doctors are not much help. My partner talked to the neuro doc who tells her there is no reason for my symptoms. That is nice. I remind myself to take it one day at a time, that tomorrow I could feel better. I thank you all for your thoughtful words and support.

Who am I and where is my life going from here

September 24, 2008 at 8:38pm—No Comments

Today, I received a call from my supervisor. She was checking on me, but changes in the center came up in conversation. I then got a call from the voc. rehab evaluation center, saying they had a cancellation and if I wanted to come this week as opposed to Oct. 19th. Yes, then it will be quicker to get back to work, if I even still have a job, then the nurse said it was too soon after my last shunt surgery. I also talked with a good friend about me wanting to work and whether going back to the same center was what I should do. I feel somewhat better since this surgery, but I still would not say the power is on or that I am me again. I want to work. I have a master's degree and several years' experience. Yet I am unclear as to what is the right way to go. I am told the VR program will be able to fully evaluate my progress and my ability to work. I have worked hard to get to the point I was at before the aneurysm, somehow the VR program feels like starting over. I want to keep an open mind. Maybe it is not meant for me to return to my old job, but who would want a 45-year-old person who just recovered from major health problems? All this keeps going through my head. I then do what I have taught many clients to do. I recite the serenity prayer and try to decide in this situation what I can control and what I can't control. I am a very capable person and somehow I will know what to do. Thanks for listening. For now, I must remember I am still Kelli and to take it one day at a time.

Feeling better today—parts of recovery

My last entry, I wasn't doing good, but today is better. This reminded me that recovery is made up of steps. I won't bore you with listing them, just know in any recovery process you have bad days and good days. One thing that helped today was being able to talk with people. You don't feel so alone when you can talk to someone, even on the phone. I got to talk to my mother and wished her a happy birthday. She was encouraging. As I have said before, laughter is a part of recovery. I get that from the *Ellen Show*, and watching reruns of the *Golden Girls*. Like my mother reminded me today, another part to recovery is patience. Of course, that is the hardest for me. Take care all and I will blog again tomorrow.

Kelli Schoen on September 28, 2008 at 5:00 pm—No Comments

Friday, I did okay but stayed home all day. Sat., Lori and I went to see the movie *Eagle Eye.* How could we not after Ellen had the actor on the show last week. I did okay and could say I was starting to feel some power coming back on. Even my vision was somewhat better. Then, today, I feel just as bad as before the shunt surgery. This all gets frustrating, but I keep fighting to continue to totally recover.

Added by Kelli Schoen on October 1, 2008 at 1:30pm—No Comments

If you don't have the courage...............

"If you don't have the courage to make a start, you have made the finish already" (author unknown). This is a quote I heard in college that has helped me throughout the years, and I find myself relying on it again. Today, Lori, my life partner, called with news from one of my neuro doctors not wanting to write me out of work more, but these are also the docs that refuse to write the okay to return to work letter I need before my job will let me come back. Then everyone, including Lori, thinks I need to go through the voc. rehab program to be evaluated as to my ability to work before going back to work. I suppose my courage to make a start in this situation is to go to the vocational rehab program. I fear me being out of work much longer will cost me my job. You see, before this job, I struggled to find a decent job in my field. I had to live in a halfway home for a time. I had help to find other types of jobs to prove I could work, so I now feel like I have gone backwards. I was doing so good until the aneurysm. If it was just me, I might push the docs to write the return to work letter. I have to keep in mind Lori. I understand her concern that if I go back too soon and get sick and how that will affect us. I just want to be better and be able to work and do the other things I enjoyed. Even though my job was not perfect, I actually miss it! I miss my co-workers and the clients I was working with.

Well, I will figure out what "start" I need to do. Remember this quote, it will help you. Have a good day.

Added by Kelli Schoen on October 4, 2008 at 5:42pm—No Comments

It's not good being me these days

I went to my GP today due to rib pain, as I thought she confirmed I had pneumonia (not spelt correct) As we talked about the struggles with the neuro doc and all the physical problems I have had, she looked at me and said, "It's not good being you, is it?" Of course, I said yep. She then said, "But we still love you." She did hit the nail on the head. It's not good being me, but I won't give up. I feel emotionally drained from all this. I don't feel I deserve good friends, good things, etc. I know it sounds bleak, but as usual I will snap out of this. I just am ready to feel normal again!

Added by Kelli Schoen on October 6, 2008 at 5:37pm—No Comments

There is a world outside my house

Today, Lori took me to the mall in Pineville, NC. It was good to get out and see people. We had to go buy Carolina Panthers stuff, even though friends would say I have plenty. If you have been reading my blogs, you know I have been through a lot lately, but I would be the first to say I know others have it worse than I do. Going out today, I was reminded there is a world outside my house. I am as guilty as others, that my drama seems so big, because we forget there is a world outside our own.

Added by Kelli Schoen on October 19, 2008 at 5:50pm—No Comments

Sunday, Oct. 19th, starts a new phase of my recovery and I'm scared as heck

Oct 19th. I begin an inpatient program in Columbia, SC, at the SC Vocational Rehabilitation Comprehensive Evaluation Center. I have been encouraged by my family doctor, my partner, and some friends that I should go to this program so that they can better evaluate what I can or cannot do as far as work, and will better prepare me to go back to work. My goal is to return to my old job, which I keep being told want me back, so this program should help me with that goal, so why am I scared?

Posted on November 4, 2008 at 10:00am—Edit Post

Made it through orientation

Today was orientation at the voc. rehab program I have come to. All the staff was very kind and encouraging. I did not get to watch the Ellen Show today, but once I find out when it is on down here, I will be advocating watching it so others can have laughter as part of their recovery. The nurses say I provide laughter myself. Well, keep smiling and have a great day.

Posted on October 20, 2008 at 4:59pm—Edit Post

Hello my name is Kelli

Today, I travelled to the VOC Rehab program. Lori brought me. Even though I am 45, I feel like a kid dropped off for camp, like a fish out of water. At my job, at home, I can hold my own in conversation and all. But in a strange environment, I have to push myself to not sit in my room and isolate.

Orientation is tomorrow. We will see how it goes. By the way, I got the laptop up for now, obviously, or would not be blogging. Smile and have a good day.

Rehab sucked, but I cannot give up.

I made it through 2 weeks and got kicked out of the voc. rehab program. My partner and I were told that my brain was not healed enough for me to be in the program. Said I needed a year from my injury date. Okay, did no one look at the medical records that were sent to know when my stroke was before accepting me into the program? They told my local VR counselor that I was emotional and unsteady on my feet. I was honest that I had one day that I got tearful because Lori kept calling needing letters from the staff here for my insurance company. It is very frustrating not being able to be in control of these things.

Posted on November 20, 2008 at 1:53pm—Edit Post

I went Bowling

Yes, I got kicked out of stroke rehab with them saying I was not healed enough, etc., but I was able to bowl 4 games with my 14 lb. balls with no problems. My high game was a 140 even. I am glad to still be alive and able to do things I want to do. Rehab kicking me out, saying I cannot do, just pissed me off and I don't give up so easily and being able to bowl and hold my own proved to me I can do. Everyone have a great day.

As thanksgiving approaches, I find myself doing a mental list of what I am thankful for. This is not easy after what I have gone through since Feb. 2008. I have lost the ability to drive, cannot work yet, and feel less independent. I can say I am thankful for having a life partner who, so far, has hung in here with me through all this. I am thankful I am above ground, I understand that was close. I am thankful I have the survivor instinct and keep plugging along toward my goals. I will not accept this is it!

Posted on November 20, 2008 at 1:53pm

Blogs off My Website

Today has been a full day. I went to my 1 p.m. brain injury therapy group, and this time, Kaci got to come along. She was so excited when I pulled out her therapy dog vest. She did so well in the group. I was so proud of her. After group, Kaci and I began our trip from Rock Hill, SC, to Moncks Corner, SC, which, depending on how heavy your foot is on the gas, is about a three-hour drive. I was so glad I was able to keep focused for that long. Since the

BI, my attention is not very good. On this trip, for example, I found my mind starting to think about other things while driving and I would have to tell myself to focus.

Tuesday, October 30, 2012

Family

Lori & I just returned from a trip to Connecticut. We were up there for about a week to visit my biological family. I have not been up to see them in about 2 years. My Mom is in her 70s so I need to be visiting her more. I don't want to be wishing I had & time had passed me by. Don't get me wrong, she is healthy & will probably outlive all of us, but you just never know. I so enjoyed seeing the family members I did get to visit with. My uncle George and his wife, who has always been my favorite uncle; my Aunt Doris, who is such a lovely lady; my cousin Kelly, who I have always felt a connection with ever since I found my family when I was in the 10th grade. My Mom showed us a nice time. I did have a hard time staying as active as she would like. She doesn't all the way get the brain being tired affecting the whole body, I think.

My only problem on this trip was that as much as I enjoyed visiting with my family, I felt disconnected. Some of that is from the brain injury, but some of that is due to the fact that we don't keep in touch as much as we could. This is a wake-up call for me that I thought I would share with you.

Don't wait until months & years go by and you feel like a stranger in your own family to realize you need to work on having better communication with them. In this day & age, you have telephones, cell phones, e-mail, Skype, and even snail mail to communicate with family members. Don't wait for them to contact you—you take the lead. It will make their day to hear from you. If you do this, you will feel closer with your family & that will help you in your recovery. I will be trying this with my family, that's for sure!

As we have been remembering 9/11 it made me think of the risk people took that day. Like the first responders going into the Trade Centers not knowing they were going to fall. Or the risk of ordinary citizens to help each other not knowing if another attack was coming. We as Americans saw huge risks being taken by our fellow Americans that day, all to help fight for survival.

This makes me think about our recovery journey and the risk we need to take to survive this journey.

4-28-2010 Update

It has been a little over 2 years since my brain 'blew up,' as I call it, and I continue to recover. I get the feeling that some people think I should "get over it" or "move on." Well, I have been trying to do both. When you have a brain injury, it will be with you the rest of your life. You just have to figure out what your life will be with the brain injury. Like I said on my profile page, I am learning to reinvent myself.

Accepting The New Me

It was about a year ago I had to accept the fact that I could not return to my job of 13 years as a Mental Health Counselor that I loved. As with many people, my job was a big part of who I was, so I have had to explore different options to help fill that void. Just recently my dog Kaci and I have begun obedience training with the hope & plan to take therapy dog training, That way, when we finish, we can volunteer doing pet therapy :). I have been working with SC VR and now am planned to begin the VR workshop on 4-25-2010.

Classes with Kaci and the workshop both are steps to help me be more active so I am glad for them. The problem is my brain is causing me some trouble. For about a month now, I have been having lightheadedness and, at times, pressure and headaches. I blame my brain, but I really don't know what is causing it, but it makes it hard to be active with that going on. I wish the doctors could put in a clinic or something and run all the tests they need to get to the bottom of this. It gets frustrating making plans and then not being able to follow through, like I had to miss one of Kaci's classes last week due to this. Thing is, though, I just won't stop planning for the future. I cannot believe that God led me to the best surgeons and professionals to save my life just to have me sit home alone all day. I know one day I will be sharing my story with others to help them.

Life Continues

It has been about a year and a half since my brain injury and I continue to recover. I attend a group for brain injury survivors. It helps to be in a room with others who understand what it is really like living with a brain injury. I receive cognitive therapy. I am just now starting to volunteer twice a week at Catawba Mental Health in the administration office. I am answering the phone and doing light clerical duties. It feels good to do this, but it saddens me to realize my brain has not recovered enough for me to return to a full-time position as a counselor. Each day, I push myself to continue with my recovery. I survived horrible events in my childhood and I will survive this. I will continue to live my life and see where I end up. I will use all I learned from my past to reinvent myself. I still want to use what

I have gone through to help others. Life continues and I continue to survive and thrive.

It is now October 2009 and I continue to recover. Since I wrote the last part in July 2009, I had a set back that reminded me yet again that recovering from a brain injury is a long, slow road to travel. August 2009, I was in the Brain Injury Program at the SC Vocational Rehabilitation Evaluation Center in Columbia, SC. This was my second time in this program, and this time I appeared to be doing well. One day, I went into a class and sat down to take a test. After the teacher handed out the test and was giving us instructions, something went wrong. My left hand drew up and I could not control it. I felt weird. I remember telling the teacher that something was wrong and hearing her calling the nurses station. The head nurse and the teacher helped me down to the nurses' station. I was so scared I was having a stroke. They called EMS and I was taken to the local hospital. My partner was called and she met me at the hospital. The ER doctor said I had a seizure. I was given an IV of Dilantin that helps with seizures but slowed me down big time. I was sent home. I was so disappointed to not be able to finish the program again, but was told when my doctors clear me I could go back. Trust me, I plan to go back and finish the program. I want their recommendations as to my work abilities.

Since coming home from that program I have had to adjust to not driving again. I was told I have to be seizure free for 6 months before I can drive again. So I ask for rides, get a cab, or walk if I can to get to where I need to go. I am even more determined to do whatever it takes to get better. The setback helped me to listen to my brain and not overdo it. Yes, I still hope to work again one day, but I must focus on getting healed and healthy first then see what is after that. One step at a time. I am more determined than ever to quit my addiction so to help with my recovery. I am a nicotine addict and I would say it probably played a part in this health issue. I attend NICA and take one day at a time. I long for the day to be free from this nasty addiction.

*As of June 19, 2010, I have not smoked a cigarette in 190 days! I can't believe it but I finally quit the nasty habit. What a miracle in itself.

Another thing I am doing to help with my recovery is to keep connected with others. With not being able to drive and money tight, it would be easy to shut off from the outside world, but that will not be helpful. That is where I had to think outside the box. We shut off the landline and increased our minutes on our cell phone plan so I could call someone during the day if need be.

I did make it through the six months of no driving and got another chance to go to the brain injury program at the SC Vocational Rehabilitation Evaluation Center in Columbia, SC. I was excited and nervous all together. I kept saying, "Third time's the charm," but I found myself having sorta flashbacks of the seizure from the last time I was there and that would scare me! I sure didn't want another seizure and not be able to drive for 6 months again. Well, I talked that fear out and put my best effort into the program. It was five weeks of physical therapy, occupational therapy, exercises, educational classes, and more, and I made it through the entire 5 weeks. I was proud of myself and my brain. The results from the evaluation were not as I hoped. They would only suggest part-time work if I was to work and not back in my old job. Basically, my memory and processing were the problems. So, I came home with no real plan. I went back to sitting around the house with my dog. I would try to make plans to take Kaci to the park or something, but not follow through. I remembered learning in Columbia that is a common problem with BI survivors, so I began to try to organize better to help me get involved with things, like helping with the local BIA support group. I tried to get everyone I knew to join Facebook and that way I could keep people posted on my status and sorta interact with people. It helped me to not feel all alone.

Depression

I have battled the old demons while going through this recovery. I find myself feeling depressed and getting down on myself. Depression is common after surviving a major medical event. A visit from Annie was enough to bring on the depression. I feared I would end up in the deep severe depression like I had in the 1990s. My self-esteem took a beating growing up, and all the negative messages seemed to come out now while I was trying to recover. I would find myself making a mistake, like losing something, and my old negative messages would want to kick in. Automatically, I may think or say "You're so stupid" or "You can't do anything right." At least now, I can automatically stop that train of thought and correct it. I may have a brain injury, but that doesn't mean I am stupid. I may have poor memory and have difficulties doing some things, but I know I can do other things well. Plus, I can be proud of what I have accomplished in my life against the odds.

Treatment

I got involved in outpatient treatment at: Carolina NeuroServices. There, I was seen by a neuropsychologist, Dr. Ewert, and occupational and physical therapists. I received services to help with my cognitive deficits, which include my memory, and also help with my depression. Dr. Ewert also had me join a therapy group that he runs for individuals recovering from brain injuries. I called us Ewert's heads one day, and it stuck. Even though we all may have different brain injuries, it has been such a great support being a part of that group. They have helped me so much. It is important that you get involved in a support group or a therapy group made up of others who have gone through a similar medical event as you. I have found they seem to understand and connect with you in a way that is really beneficial.

During this time, I also continued to work with my vocational rehabilitation counselor to try to ready myself for employment. We decided to try working at the VR Training Workshop. It is a training site to help evaluate and prepare people for employment. I had sent clients there in the past. Never thought I'd be going there, but I had to start somewhere. At this point, I had been out of work and unproductive for a little over two years. The first day at the workshop was a humbling experience. I ran into not one but two ex-clients that I kind of worked with on my job at Mental Health, both in crisis situations. I assured them I would not share that with anyone, and I didn't. I fit in okay with my co-workers. The jobs were production jobs. One job I had was to put 4 screws into a plastic bag. Later, I would be assigned to seal the bags. I never minded any job I was assigned, but it was obvious that I was much slower than the other workers. I would catch myself thinking, *"What are you doing? You have a master's degree and you are now at this level and can't do it well."* I then would recite the serenity prayer or my favorite quote: "The person who lacks the courage to make a start has made the finish already." That would get me back on track and help me remember that it was only a stepping-stone toward my goal to work one day. Being slow was a problem that one of the supervisors pointed out one day. This would frustrate me because as with any job I have had, I wanted to be good at it. But with my brain injury, I didn't move as quick, and my left-side neglect syndrome really caused problems with moving fast using the left hand. My biggest problem working at the workshop was the fatigue it was causing. My VR counselor came out to the workshop on the second week to check on me, and before I could say a word, she said I looked worn out. We tried cutting my hours back but my brain was still getting fatigued. I talked to my main brain doctors, Dr. W and Dr. Ewert, and we agreed that I should discontinue the workshop at that time. I would work on my occupational and cognitive therapies and start my therapy dog training with my dog Kaci and do some volunteering.

Therapy Dog Training

I got Kaci about 6 months before Annie's arrival, and she was about two or three months old then, so she has grown up with me recovering. I say she has been my 24/7 therapy dog. It only made sense when my first OT, Julie, suggested we get trained to do pet therapy to do it! So I got on the internet and found an organization in my area, Highland Canine, which provided therapy dog training. I made the arrangements, and in June 2010, Kaci and I began therapy dog training. Every Tuesday evening, we would get in the car and head to Matthews, North Carolina, to the home of Linda Taylor, our trainer. Kaci looked forward to these classes. It was good for her to learn what she was learning, but to be around other dogs was good too. It scared me to death at times. I was bitten by a German shepherd as a child, so I fear big dogs. Linda had German shepherds and there were a couple other big dogs in the class. So, if there was a bark fest my anxiety went through the roof! However, I would not allow this to stop me from getting my therapy dog training. I believed Kaci and I made a great pet therapy team. I wouldn't give up on that goal. While I wasn't working on that, I have started being the facilitator for the BIA Support Group in Rock Hill. Since my brain injury was on the right side of my brain, the left side is still intact. That means my education and work experience were still there as well as my long-term memories. So, when it was made known to me that the group needed a facilitator, I thought maybe I should give it a try. No, it's not like having my old job back, but it allowed me to help others, so I began doing that. The meetings were only once a month. I just sent out reminder e-mails and was the contact person for the group, etc. I also got the idea that I could volunteer speaking, sharing my story if an organization, church, etc., so desired. I began in June 2010 telling people I was available, calling or visiting organizations I thought might use such service. I was starting to get excited about the possibilities of my future.

Writings

Throughout my life I used writing as a way to cope with life. I have decided to share with you some of those writings. You will get a sense of what I was feeling and how I was dealing with life at the time of the writing.

Turn the Lights On (April 2008)

Someone please turn the lights back on. It appears we have a power failure. That is how it feels in my head since 02-06-08. On that day, I had a brain aneurysm rupture and hemorrhaged in my brain. I am told I am lucky to be alive. I am told just how far I have come so far in my recovery. Today, I can see this, but this does not change how I or my brain feels. I try hard to accept where I am right now. I am thankful I can walk and use both my arms. The only real deficit that prevents me from driving, working, and being independent is vision problem in my left eye. This change in my daily functioning has led to depression, which seems to add to the feeling that the power is off and I have no lights. It may not sound like a big deal, but it is hard to move without power. I try to accept my brain and myself, but it is hard to forget all I had accomplished up to that day and now the lights are out. The best way to explain this so you can understand what I am trying to say is imagine that you are in your home at night and a horrible storm comes up that knocks out the power to your home. You have your home, you know where things are, but without power you are limited as to what you can do. No lights to see clearly, no microwave for popcorn, etc. That is how it is with my brain feeling like lights are out. I want to drive, work, bowl; I want friends that I can spend time with and truly be there, not deadhead. I am thankful to be alive, but I need the power turned back on so I can live my life.

How Am I? (June 2010)

I am asked "How you doing?" and I usually reply with "Okay" or "All right" and that usually gets me by. Do you really want to know how I am? I don't think you do so I don't go in to it. You don't want to know that everyday is a challenge these days. One minute I can feel half way decent and then out of nowhere my brain begins to feel like someone is filling it up with added air. Kinda feels like a beer buzz but without the fun of drinking with your buddies, and along with that problem I am having numbness or tingling in parts of my body on and off. You don't want to know I get so scared when I get a migraine, that the pain makes me worry about the possibility of my brain blowing up again. You don't want to know that since the brain injury, I don't feel emotionally the same and I worry sometimes how that affects my interactions with other people, especially my friends and my partner. You don't really want to know that I am still feeling like I have woken up in another person's life and I'm just quietly trying to fit in. You probably don't want to know about the times I think of how I can use this brain injury event to help others, to have that taken out of my memory banks as soon as I quit thinking about it and making me realize I'm a dreamer and how useless I feel. You don't want to know that I am feeling alone, that my old friends are gone. Oh sure, if I pick up the phone and call one of them, they would try to talk with me but it's been over a year since any of them have called me. I know it's because they don't know what to say but I am still alone.

Finally, you don't want to know how tired I am of the ups and downs of this brain injury recovery and wish there was some way to take a break, but I can't leave my brain. We need each other to survive. So, I must continue on. I will continue on.

The Split

I had lost a lot due to Annie, but I continued trying to remain positive. I needed to do that to help me continue to move forward in my recovery journey. So, when I was told I couldn't work, I found a way to volunteer that wouldn't tax my brain. I had a hard time in October 20011 though. It was then that Lori, my life partner at that time, and I decided it was in our best interest to split up and go our separate ways. This was so hard to come to that decision. We had been together for almost ten years.

The problem was—as I see it, that is—I was not the same person since Annie, and some of the changes really affected Lori. One in particular was I had no sex drive. There were other changes as well. I just wasn't the same since Annie came to visit me. Lori was trying to understand. I am so grateful that she stuck by me as long as she did. I know that it wasn't easy. I realized she wasn't happy and I was feeling guilty that I had changed and could not change back. I was feeling guilty that Lori was so unhappy, and when she admitted it during a talk we had in mid October 2011, I admitted I wasn't happy either. Because she was unhappy, Lori was tense a lot and would be fussy at home. I learned to not to take it personally.

Well, no split up goes perfect now, does it? We had to get the house cleaned out to sell. This meant we would have to remain living together in the same house. This was not that easy. Lori wanted to remain in control of my finances. I had to dig down deep inside me to get my guts to stand up and take control of my finances back. I was proud of that! Now, remember, Lori had to be over everything. I was not able to take care of my financial matters, but now I was getting better and I was able to convince Lori I needed control back. I was nervous talking to her about it. You see, Annie somehow took my self-esteem. I had to start over in that area also.

Thanksgiving 2011 was lonely. Lori left Wednesday night to go to her parents. I remained at home with Kaci. I could have gone with Lori, but I just did not feel like it. I thought it would feel awkward. I felt I needed to get used to being alone anyhow.

Out on My Own

March 9, 2012

I moved out on my own into a two-bedroom apartment. I had mixed emotions about this; I was sad because it was truly the end of my ten-year relationship with Lori, yet I was excited too because I had recovered well enough from Annie that I could live on my own. I know that this doesn't always happen! I am very fortunate, so I was happy to be able to move into my apartment with my dog and cat.

Living on my own was taxing on my brain at first. I found myself being more fatigued the first couple months. I figured it was because I was doing more; just being more in charge of my life. I tried to organize my apartment in hopes to keep me organized. See, since Annie, I have learned I needed to be organized to minimize confusion in my life. I even tried to set up a system to help me with paying bills. For the most part, the system has helped.

Living on my own actually helped me as I was learning to accept the new me.

The New Me

When Annie arrived, the old Kelli went away. Sometimes, that still makes me feel sad, except at this point, I'm not sure I remember much about old Kelli. The one difference I do remember is old Kelli was free spirited. Relaxed. Since Annie came to visit, I don't feel as relaxed or free spirited. I do miss that!

I am learning to accept the new me. I accept that my brain doesn't operate like it used to. Adjusting to the blind spot in my vision. Adjusting to not being able to get up and go into the office. That has been the hardest thing to adjust to. When I released myself from the idea of returning to my job, to my surprise, there was a sense of relief over me.

I found the more I was able to let go of trying to be the old Kelli, I was better able to accept the New Me!

Running

Living on my own was stressful on my brain at times. I would release some of that stress with my running. That's right, I said running. Before Annie came to visit me, I was a runner. In college, I ran 10K races for fun. At first, Dr. W wasn't so sure about letting me run. I had to explain to him that I ran before the injury. I also told him I researched on the internet and found other stroke survivors who ran after they had strokes. Sometimes, you have to fight for what you want. Once I did get cleared by Dr. W to run, I began slowly working my way to where I could run around the neighborhood. I had to keep in mind that my body needed time to work up to any distance. I do hope to do 5K or 10K one day. I am happy that Annie didn't take running from me.

Lessons from Annie

I have mentioned that Annie has taken things from me. Like my job! Yes! Annie has taken from me but I have also learned so much since Annie's visit. My first lesson from Annie was patience, something anyone who is recovering from any major medical event has to learn. I have always been an overachiever, and so it made sense I expected myself to heal and get back in my life. Every time I was told recovering from a brain injury was a long and slow process, I wanted to believe I would be different. Finally, I got the message! I began to be patient with myself. I listened to what my brain was telling me. If it needed to rest, I rested and tried to not feel bad about doing nothing. I learned I had to give my brain the time to recover.

Annie has taught me to slow down! Boy, I wish I had learned this lesson so many years ago! I was the type of person that went into the office and worked through lunch most of the time. I was all about my job. Don't get me wrong, I loved my job! I think I just needed to pace myself better than I did then.

Annie has taught me life is short. I need to enjoy what I have of it!

It has been four years and six months since Annie came to visit me. She sure did turn my life upside down! Nothing looks the same. During this time, I remember my favorite quote—"The person who lacks the courage to make a start has made the finish already,"—to keep me going forward.

I am learning recovery from Annie is a continuous journey. People seem to look at me oddly when I remark that I'm recovering from a brain injury and share what happened. They seem to expect I'm talking about a TBI (traumatic brain injury) and they seem surprised at the amount of time that has passed. I pay them no attention. I still struggle with myself from time to time with the fact that my brain has not healed enough for me to work. So, I can see how it can be hard for people to understand that recovering from a brain injury is not like recovering from a broken bone.

I think that maybe, because the brain is like the motherboard of our entire body—if it goes down, other things don't work so well—when the wires do get crossed, it takes time to reprogram them. This is just how I've come to understand it. Remember, I'm just an aneurysm/stroke survivor! I have no medical knowledge.

I know the recovery journey I am on has been long, and it will continue. I have had some bumps in the road on this journey. You have those when you are recovering from a major medical event. That is no reason to give up! I figured I survived Annie and the stroke! I need to do what is necessary to live my life!

It really has to do with your thinking. There have been days that I would feel so down and use negative thinking. It was the ability to switch the negative thinking into positive thoughts that got me through. For example, every time I began to think, "I had to give up living in a house with a fenced-in yard," I got where I would counter that thought with, "I'm living in a nice apartment that I would have never been able to afford if I didn't work for the state all those years before Annie." I hate that Annie had to come and visit me, but I choose to make it into a positive by sharing this with you. Remember, don't give up! Remember my favorite quote: "The person who lacks the courage to make a start has made the finish already." You are not finished! Take it at your pace and ask for help when you need it. You are the only one that can truly push yourself while you are on your recovery journey. If you have cheerleaders, that is great! I sure did, but when it comes down to really pushing yourself, that is up to you!

I hope sharing my visit from Annie will be of help to you on your journey. Remember to believe in yourself and do not give up!